Renal Diet Mastery

Low Sodium, Low Potassium Recipes For The Newly Diagnosed To Managing Kidney Diseases And Avoiding Dialysis

David Lawrence

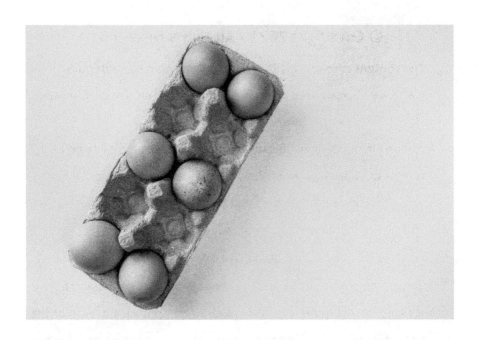

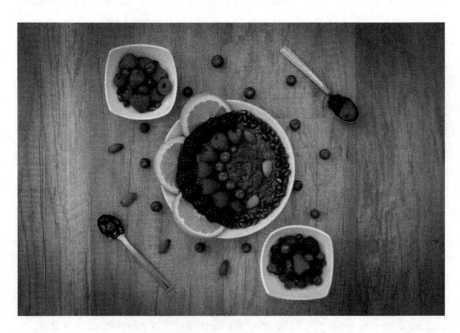

Table of Contents

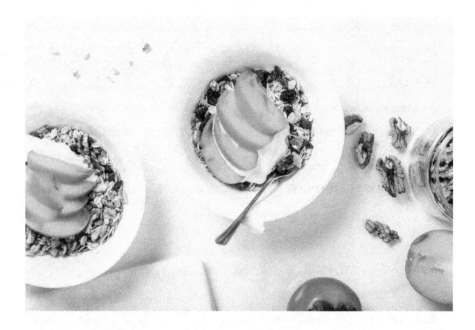

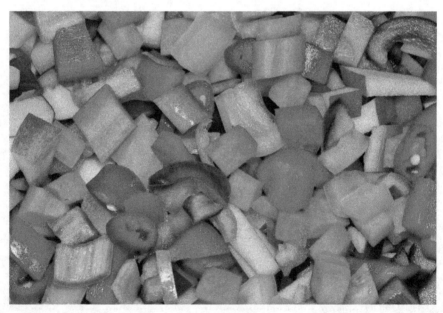

Introduction

The renal diet is a diet that is prescribed to diabetic patients to control their urine output. You must know the term of the renal diet so that you can follow this diet and can be easily controlled for the betterment of diabetic problems.

Normally the kidney of any patient is not functioning as per the requirement, it is working below the requirement, and this lack of function is very dangerous for the body in fact and can even result in drastic changes in the kidneys. In short, it is known as renal failure. The people who are suffering from this problem must have a proper check-up to know the extent of the problem. If a proper check is done, it can be easily detected.

So, therefore, it is better to know about what the renal diet is and how to do it, how to cure the disease, and how to make the kidney work properly?

Renal diet is also known as "Diabetic diet." As the kidney of a diabetic patient is not working properly, this diet helps to control the urine output of the diabetic patient. So this diet is very useful in case of an accidental patient. Although the patient has diabetes, still doctor will recommend him/her to do this diet. This diet helps to control the amount of sugar that is excreted in the urine. By controlling the urine sugar excretion, the patient can have fewer complications caused by diabetes.

According to some specialists, the renal diet is very useful in diabetic patients only. A patient who is suffering from cancer, kidney disease, heart disease, lung disease must not follow a renal diet as it will weaken his physical condition, and he may not be able to recover from the diseases properly. But before going for this diet, everyone should consult with the doctor.

The special thing about the renal diet is in the kind of food which is good for healthy kidneys. In normal cases, if a person is suffering from some disease, but if he has a proper diet then he can easily recover. If there is some deficiency in the kidney, there is some problem with this kidney cannot work properly for all the people, some people can be able to work properly. But the problem of the kidney will be very severe due to diabetes.

The kidney is a place where a lot of waste, purifies and extracts all the waste and impurities from the body. It is a very important organ of the human body. If this organ does not work properly, the body will not be able to function properly.

Foods to be eaten and foods not to be eaten are as follows:

- Foods included in renal diet

- Food category foods to be included.

- Rice, wheat, bajra, maize, supa, fusals.

- Milk, curd, buttermilk.

- Toast, idli, dosa, chapati, puri, kachori, bhakri, paratha.

- All kinds of pulses.

- All kinds of vegetables except tomato and brinjal.

- Sweet dishes (gulab jamun, fried bread, halwa, pakoda, curdi, rasgula, etc.)

- Sweets, kulfi, peda, etc.

- Jaggery and its candies.

- Sugar, salt, ghee.

- All kinds of condiments and spice.

- Dried fruit and nuts.

- Nuts like cashew, coconut, peanuts.

- Ghee, oil, gingelly, turmeric.

- Coconut meat and milk.

- Any kind of fish.

- Any kind of meat.

- Tofu.

- Boiled potatoes, boiled sweet potatoes, boiled white potatoes,

- Anything which is fried.

- Any kind of vegetable made of wheat flour.

- Whole wheat, rye, oat.

- Foods that must not be eaten

- Helps to control the urine output

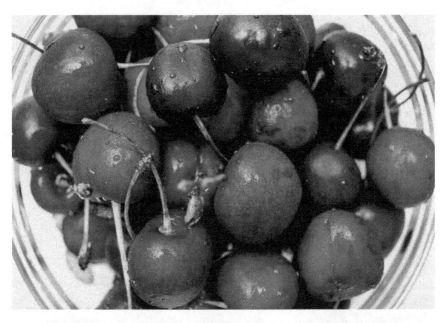

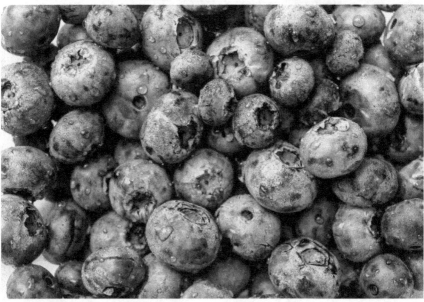

Chapter 1:

The Renal Diet

Stages

In this case, kidney disease is a chronic condition (CKD) where the kidneys fail gradually to do their normal job. Chronic kidney disease typically develops in 5 stages. Each stage is measured by a formula called Glomerular Filtration Rate (GFR), calculated by several variables like age, race, gender, and serum creatinine in the urine. The higher this protein is in the system, the more progressed the renal disease stage will be. Here is a brief snapshot of each stage.

- **Stage 1**: considered the normal or high risk of developing CKD. The GFR falls > 90 mL/min.

- **Stage 2**: considered as mild CKD. The GFR falls in the range of 60–89 mL/min.

- **Stage 3:** Moderate CKD, which ranges from 45–59 mL/min.

- **Stage 4:** Severe Chronic Kidney disease. Rates fall between 15–29 mL/min.

- **Stage 5:** Final/end-stage of the renal disease, which calls for surgery or dialysis. Also called End-Stage Renal Disease (ESRD). The GFR levels, in this case, fall below 15 mL/min.

Causes

Now, in regards to the actual causes or risk factors that may contribute to the formation of disease, studies have indicated the following conditions:

- **Diabetes.** Diabetes is probably the No.1 cause of renal disease as the bloodstream's increased blood glucose can ruin blood vessels inside the kidneys.

- **Heart disease.** Heart disease has also been found to have a negative association with CKD. Those with chronic heart problems, in particular, have a higher probability of developing the renal disease as well.

- **Elevated blood pressure.** Abnormally high blood pressure can ruin the kidneys' delicate blood vessels and make them function poorly as a result.

- **Genetic History of Renal Disease.** If any of your family members and especially parents and grandparents have already developed the disease, there is a higher chance of developing it. If any of your family members has kidney disease, it would be wise to get tested too and encourage other family members to do the same.

In addition to the above common causes, autoimmune disorders like Lupus and nephrotic syndrome can increase renal disease risk. Also, urinary problems and certain medications, e.g., diuretics or antibiotics, as well as illegal drugs, can interfere with the normal function of the kidneys and cause damage. For this reason, consult your doctor for medication.

Symptoms

The disease's problem is that it often comes with little or no symptoms at all, especially during the first stages. You may experience the following symptoms, but these could also be a sign of another condition:

- Less frequent urination.

- A very little amount of urine.

- Sudden and unexplained pauses in breath.

- Nausea.

- Chest or back pain.

- Drowsiness and dizziness.

- Dry skin, itchy skin.

- Fatigue/feeling tired more than before.

- Confusion.

- Loss of balance.

- Muscle cramps, especially at night.

- Swelling in the face, ankles, feet, and hands.

- Poor appetite.

Diagnosis

Your family doctor can prescribe two tests:

Blood Test

Glomerular filtration rate (GFR) and serum creatinine level. Creatinine is one of those end products of protein metabolism. The blood level depends on age, gender, muscle mass, nutrition, physical activity, and foods before taking the sample (for example, a lot of meat was eaten), and some drugs. Creatinine is expelled from the body through the kidneys, and if the work of the kidneys slows down, the creatinine levels present in the blood plasma rises. Determining the creatinine level alone is insufficient for diagnosing chronic kidney disease since its value begins to exceed the upper limit of the norm only when GFR decreases by half. To calculate GFR, you include four parameters into your formula that take into account the creatinine reading, age, gender, and race of the patient. GFR shows at what level is the ability of the kidneys to filter. In the case of chronic kidney disease, the GFR indicator shows the stage of the severity of kidney disease.

Urine Analysis

The content of albumin in the urine is determined; also, the values of albumin and creatinine in the urine are determined by each other. Albumin is a protein in the urine that usually enters the urine in minimal quantities. Even a small increase in the level of albumin in the urine in some people may be an early sign of incipient kidney disease, especially in those with diabetes and high blood pressure. In the case of normal kidney function, albumin in the urine should be no more than 3 mg/mmol (or 30 mg/g). If albumin excretion increases even more, then it already speaks of kidney disease. If albumin excretion exceeds 300 mg/g, other proteins are excreted into the urine, and this condition is called proteinuria.

- If the kidney is healthy, then albumin does not enter the urine.

- In the case of an injured kidney, albumin begins to enter the urine.

- If the doctor suspects that there is a kidney disease after receiving the urine analysis results, then an additional urine analysis is performed for albumin. If albuminuria or proteinuria is detected again within three months, then this indicates chronic kidney disease.

Nutrients You Need

Potassium

Potassium is a mineral found in nearly all foods in varying amounts. Our bodies need an amount of potassium to help with muscle activity as well as electrolyte balance and regulation of blood pressure. However, if potassium is in excess within the system and the kidneys can't expel it (due to renal disease), fluid retention and muscle spasms can occur.

Phosphorus

Phosphorus is a trace mineral found in many foods, especially dairy, meat, and eggs. It acts synergistically with calcium as well as vitamin D to promote bone health. However, when there is damage in the kidneys, excess amounts of the mineral cannot be taken out, causing bone weakness.

Calories

When being on a renal diet, it is vital to give yourself the right number of calories to fuel your system. It depends on your age, gender, general health status, and renal disease stage the exact number of calories you should take. In most cases, there are no strict limitations in the calorie intake, as long as you take them from proper sources that are low in sodium, potassium, and phosphorus. In general, doctors recommend a daily limit between 1800–2100 calories per day to keep weight within the normal range.

Protein

Protein is an essential nutrient that our systems need to develop and generate new connective tissue, e.g., muscles, even during injuries. Protein also helps stop bleeding and supports the immune system to fight infections. A healthy adult with no kidney disease would usually need 40–65 grams of protein per day.

However, in the renal diet, protein consumption is a tricky subject as too much or too little can cause problems. Protein, when being metabolized by our systems, also creates waste, which is typically processed by the kidneys. But when kidneys are damaged or underperforming, as in kidney disease, waste will stay in the system. This is why patients in more advanced CKD stages are advised to limit their protein consumption as well.

Fats

Our systems need fats and particularly good fats as a fuel source and for other metabolic cell functions. A diet rich in bad and trans or saturated fats can significantly raise the odds of developing heart problems, often with renal disease. This is why most physicians advise their renal patients to follow a diet that contains a decent amount of good fats and a meager amount of trans (processed) or saturated fat.

Sodium

Sodium (NA) is an essential mineral that our bodies need to regulate fluid and electrolyte balance. It also plays a role in normal cell division in the muscles and nervous system. However, in kidney disease, sodium can quickly spike at higher than normal levels, and the kidneys will be unable to expel it, causing fluid accumulation as a side-effect. Those who also suffer from heart problems as well should limit its consumption as it may raise blood pressure.

Carbohydrates

Carbs act as a major and quick fuel source for the body's cells. When we consume carbs, our systems turn them into glucose and then into energy for "feeding" our body cells. Carbs are generally not restricted in the renal diet. Still, some types of carbs contain dietary fiber as well, which helps regulate normal colon function and protect blood vessels from damage.

Dietary Fiber

Fiber is an important element in our system that cannot be properly digested but plays a key role in the regulation of our bowel movements and blood cell protection. The fiber in the renal diet is generally encouraged as it helps loosen up the stools, relieve constipation and bloating and protect from colon damage. However, many patients don't get enough amounts of dietary fiber per day, as many of them are high in potassium or phosphorus. Fortunately, some good dietary fiber sources for CKD patients have lower amounts of these minerals compared to others.

Vitamins/Minerals

According to medical research, our systems need at least 13 vitamins and minerals to keep our cells fully active and healthy. However, patients with renal disease are more likely to be depleted by water-soluble vitamins like B-complex and Vitamin C as a result of limited fluid consumption. Therefore, supplementation with these vitamins, along with a renal diet program, should help cover any possible vitamin deficiencies. Supplementation of fat-soluble vitamins like vitamins A, K, and E may be avoided as they can quickly build-up in the system and turn toxic.

Fluids

When you are in an advanced stage of renal disease, fluid can quickly build-up and lead to problems. While it is important to keep your system well hydrated, you should avoid minerals like potassium and sodium, which can trigger further fluid build-up and cause a host of other symptoms.

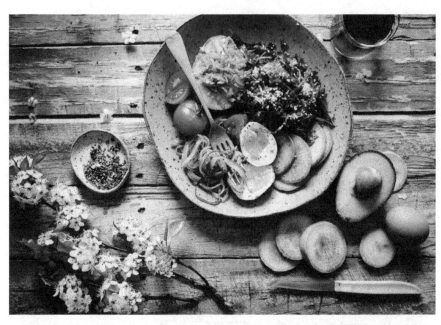

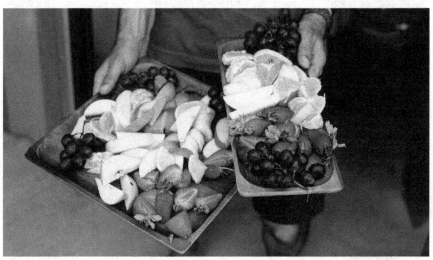

Chapter 2:

Differences between CKD and PKD in Kidney Disease

What Is a Chronic Kidney Disease?

During this hectic time of diagnosis and management of your new lifestyle, it helps explore Chronic Kidney Disease (CKD) and outline a few common symptoms. CKD can be defined simply as the gradual loss of kidney function. Since the body is constantly producing waste, the kidneys play a key role in removing these toxins and keeping your system functioning properly. Tests can be done to measure the specific level of waste in your blood and determine your kidneys' level of function. Your doctor can determine your kidney's filtration rate and identify your CKD stage based on this measurement.

Five Stages of CKD

There are five stages associated with CKD that correspond to how well your kidneys are functioning. People often do not experience any symptoms during the early stages, and the disease can be very manageable. Kidney disease can even go undetected until it is quite advanced. Many symptoms do not begin to appear until the later stages when toxins begin to build up in the body from damage to the kidneys. For example, itching, swelling, nausea, vomiting, or changes in urine patterns may result from these organs' decreased filtration ability. That's why early diagnosis is so crucial and can result in very positive outcomes concerning the disease's progression.

What Is a Renal Diet?

The renal diet is a dietary regimen designed to convey respite to patients with deliberate or injured renal functions and chronic kidney diseases. As we have already mentioned, there is no single uniformed type of renal diet—this is the case because requirements of the renal diet and restrictions need to match the patient's needs and be based on what the doctor prescribed for the patient's overall health.

However, all forms of renal diet have one thing in common: to improve your renal functions, bring some relief to your kidneys, and prevent kidneys disease in patients with numerous risk factors, altogether improving your overall health and well-being. The grocery list we have provided should help you get hold of which groceries you should introduce to your diet and which groups of food should be avoided to improve your kidneys' performance, so you can start from shopping for your new lifestyle.

You don't need to shop for many different types of groceries all at once, as it is always better to use fresh produce. However, frozen food also makes a good alternative when fresh fruit and vegetables are not available.

Remember to treat canned goods as suggested and recommended in the portion and drain excess liquid from the canned food.

For the renal diet recommended in our guide, this form of kidney-friendly dietary regimen offers a solution in the form of low-sodium and low-potassium meals and groceries, which is why we are also offering simple and easy renal diet recipes. This dietary plan is compiled for all renal system failure stages unless the doctor recommends a different treatment by allowing or expelling some of the groceries that we have listed in our ultimate grocery list for renal patients.

Before you start cooking and changing your lifestyle from the very core with the idea of improving your health, we want you to get familiar with renal diet basics. You can also find out exactly what this diet is based on, as it will help you improve your kidney health by reducing your sodium and potassium intake.

The best way of getting familiar with the renal diet and the basics of this dietary regimen is to look at the commonly asked questions.

The Effects of Renal Diet on Kidney Disease

Although there is no cure for CKD, this disease is completely manageable. Implementing changes to your diet and lifestyle may help slow the disease's development and evade symptoms that naturally begin to occur as the disease advances. These diet and regimen variations can even advance your general health and help you manage associated conditions. As we will explore in the next few portions, associated diseases may have led to CKD or perhaps were a contributing factor. When you begin making changes to your food and daily habits, you will also notice an improvement in these associated conditions, including hypertension and diabetes.

It is probable to live a long, healthy, and happy life while managing this disease. Making proper changes early on can slow the progression of any adverse symptoms for several years. I hope this book will shed this important light on you and your loved ones, so together you can make positive changes that delay the progression of CKD for a long time to come.

- **Stage 1:** Slight kidney damage, and usually no symptoms. (eGFR > 90 mL)

- **Stage 2:** Mild damage in kidneys (eGFR = 60–89 mL)

- **Stage 3:** Moderate damage in kidneys (eGFR = 30–59 mL)

- **Stage 4:** Severe damage in kidneys (eGFR = 15–29 mL)

- **Stage 5:** Kidney failure/End-stage CKD (GFR < 15 mL)

How to Manage and Improve Kidney Health

Patients who struggle with kidney health issues, going through a kidney dialysis, and having renal impairments need to go through medical treatment and change their eating habits and lifestyle to make the situation better. Many studies have been made on this. The conclusion is that food has a lot to do with how your kidney functions and its overall health.

The first thing to changing your lifestyle is knowing how your kidney functions and how different foods can trigger different kidney function reactions. Certain nutrients affect your kidney directly. Nutrients like sodium, protein, phosphate, and potassium are the risky ones. You cannot omit them altogether from your diet, but you need to limit or minimize their intake as much as possible. You cannot leave out essential nutrients like protein from your diet, but you need to count how much protein you are having per day. This is essential to keep balance in your muscles and maintaining a good functioning kidney.

A profound change in kidney patients is measuring how much fluid they are drinking. This is a crucial change in every kidney patient, and you must adapt to this new eating habit. Too much water or any other form of liquid can disrupt your kidney function. How much fluid you can consume depends on the condition of your kidney.

Chapter 3:

Overview of the Role and Use of Sodium, Potassium, Phosphorus, and Other Nutrients

G iven that you decide to accept it, your mission is to ensure that you minimize waste build-up in your kidneys. To do that, you need to watch what you eat, carefully preparing or arranging your meals so that you receive the required nutrition, minus all the unnecessary components.

This is where a renal diet becomes an essential component of your life.

Before delving deeper into the diet itself, let us look at some of the important substances that people with CKD need to manage.

Sodium

Suppose you have been enjoying your pasta, nachos, pizzas, juicy steaks, lip-smacking burgers or practically any of your favorite savory food items. In that case, the chances are that you have been consuming sodium. Why? Well, this mineral is commonly found in salt. Whether you use table salt or sea salt, you are going to find sodium in them. If you have heard people claim that sodium is harmful to your body, let me tell you that it is not entirely true. We need sodium in our bodies. The mineral helps our body maintain a balance in the levels of water within and around our cells. At the same time, it also maintains your blood pressure levels. Surprised? You might have thought that sodium makes things worse, but there is a medical condition called hyponatremia, or "low blood sodium." When sodium levels drop to a low enough level, then you experience all the symptoms below:

- Weakness.

- Nausea.

- Vomiting.

- Fatigue or low energy.

- Headache.

- Irritability.

- Muscle cramps or spasms.

- Confusion.

In conclusion, sodium is essential for your body, but when you are on a renal diet, you control the amount of salt that you add to your food. Since the kidneys are rather sensitive at this point, there is no need to exacerbate their condition by adding more sodium.

This might prove difficult for people since they are used to having salt as a flavoring ingredient in their foods. But that is why we will use recipes full of flavors that you will enjoy (more on that when we get started on the recipes).

Potassium

Potassium is considered a mineral that people might not think about too much compared to calcium or sodium, but it nonetheless serves an important role in our body.

Apart from regulating fluids, it also aids the body in passing messages between the body and the brain. Just like sodium, potassium is classified as an electrolyte, a term used to refer to a family of minerals that react in water. When potassium is dissolved in water, it produces positively charged ions and using these ions; potassium can conduct electricity, which allows it to carry out some incredibly important functions. Take, for example, the messages that are communicated between the brain and the body. These messages are sent back and forth in the form of impulses. But one has to wonder; what exactly creates those impulses? It's not like our body has an inbuilt electrical generator. The answer lies in the ions. We have already established that sodium and potassium are both electrolytes and produce ions. The impulses are created when sodium ions move into the cells, and potassium ions move out of the cell. This movement changes the voltage of the cell, producing impulses. The way the impulses are created is similar to Morse code but takes place much faster (it has to for your body to react, manage processes, or perform tasks). When the level of potassium falls, the body's ability to generate nerve impulses gets affected. Wait a minute. So potassium is good. Does that mean I am asking you to let your body give up on normal nerve impulses to keep your kidneys safe? Is that the only choice? That's a tough choice to make!

Relax. What we should do is avoid having too much potassium.

When the kidneys are not functioning properly, then their potassium build-up could cause problems to the heart. More specifically, they could change the heartbeats' rhythm, leading to a potential heart attack. But don't worry. This does not happen with just a mild increase in potassium. There has to be a significant increase to cause such a devastating result. Nevertheless, we are going to avoid even reaching a 'mild' increase. I placed the mild in quotes because there is no actual benchmark to gauge if the potassium content in your blood is mild or potentially life-threatening. It all depends on various factors in the body. I shall list down a few foods that are high in potassium that you should watch out for:

- Melons such as cantaloupe and honeydew (watermelon is acceptable).

- Oranges and orange juice.

- Winter squash.

- Pumpkin.

- Bananas.

- Prune juice.

- Grapefruit juice.

- Dried beans—all kinds.

Try to avoid granola bars (even though they are advertised as nutritious) and bran cereals.

Phosphorus

Finally, we have phosphorus. This mineral makes up about 1% of your body weight. That may not seem like a lot in actuality, but remember that our body consists of a lot of water. For this reason, oxygen makes up 62% of our total body weight, followed by carbon at 18%, hydrogen at 9%, and nitrogen at 3%. But, what are the next two main elements of the human body?

- Calcium at 1.5%.

- Phosphorus at 1%.

So you see, even though phosphorus makes up just 1% of the total body weight, it is still a significant element.

What Is It Used for?

Let me put it this way. Phosphorus is one of the reasons you can smile wide. It is the reason your skin and other parts of the body are the way they are and do not just fall on the floor, like the way a piece of cloth might when you drop it. Phosphorus is responsible for forming your teeth and the bones that keep your body structure the way it currently is.

Pretty fantastic, isn't it? We often nominate calcium as the main element in the formation of teeth and bones but forget the less popular and often overlooked partner element that helps with the same task.

However, the fact that phosphorus keeps our teeth and bones healthy is something people eventually discover. They don't discover that phosphorus also plays an important role in helping the body use fats and carbohydrates. The mineral is truly important for the everyday function of the body.

When kidney problems strike us, we don't need the extra amount of phosphorus. While phosphorus is truly important for our bones and teeth, an excessive amount in the blood can lead to weaker bones. Since most of the food we eat already includes phosphorus, we will try and avoid anything with a high mineral percentage.

Fluids

Water sustains us. After all, 60% of the human adult's body is composed of water. This is why you might have heard of popular recommendations on how you should be having about eight glasses of water per day.

There is still a debate on exactly how much water is needed by an individual daily. But the fact remains; we need enough to avoid dehydration and keep the body functioning normally.

When you have kidney disease, you may not need as much fluid as you did before. This is because damaged kidneys do not dispose of extra fluids as well as they should. All the extra fluid in your body could be dangerous. It could cause swelling in various areas, high blood pressure, and heart problems. Fluid can also build up around your lungs, preventing you from breathing normally.

There is no measurement of how much fluid is considered as extra fluid. I strongly suggest that you should visit the doctor and get more information about fluid retention from him or her. The doctor will guide you better and help you understand how much fluids you might require. The thing to understand here is that many of the foods that we eat, including fruits, vegetables, and most soups, have a water content in them as well. Getting to know your kidney's ability to hold on to fluids will help you prepare or plan better meals for yourself.

The Renal Diet

When we follow the renal diet, we are going to make use of all the information about various components and minerals of foods to prepare a meal that is as ideal for your body as possible. One of the renal diet's main aims is to manage sodium, potassium, and phosphorus intake. Simultaneously, the renal diet focuses on consuming high-quality protein and limiting the consumption of fluids. Knowing about what you should eat and what you shouldn't go a long way in finding out if there is anything in particular that you should avoid (due to allergies, for example).

Benefits of the Renal Diet

So how exactly does the renal diet benefit you?

Preventing Diabetes and High Blood Pressure from Worsening

When you manage two of the biggest contributors of CKD, you are greatly delaying the effects of the disease. You are getting out of a loop where either diabetes or high blood pressure makes the disease worse, further worsening either of the two conditions, which results in the disease entering a worse phase, and on it goes. This loop continues until it results in complete kidney failure.

Additionally, you might notice that your daily life becomes affected by CKD if you do not manage the disease. You might find yourself losing focus on the things that you like, becoming less productive, and feeling too lethargic. You might also experience a greater degree of discomfort or exhaustion, even if you only have been walking at a normal pace.

A renal diet helps you avoid all the complications of diabetes and high blood pressure daily. You might not feel as though your life has taken a heavy toll through careful planning because of the disease. You need to bring back as much normality as possible in your life, and a renal diet helps you with that.

Prevents Cardiovascular Problems

Because a renal diet manages various aspects of our health, including the consumption of sodium, potassium, and phosphorus, it aids in preventing cardiovascular risk factors from developing (Cupisti, Aparicio & Barsotti, 2007). When you manage the sodium content in your body, you also ensure that cholesterol levels are low. When you have too much cholesterol in your blood, it tends to accumulate in your arteries' walls. This process is called atherosclerosis and is a type of heart disease.

Chapter 4:

Breakfast

1. Apple-Chai Smoothie

Preparation time: 35 minutes.

Cooking time: 5 minutes.

Servings: 2

Ingredients:

- 1 cup unsweetened rice milk

- 1 chai tea bag

- 1 apple, peeled, cored, and chopped

- 2 cups ice

Directions:

1. In a medium saucepan, heat the rice milk over low heat for about 5 minutes or until steaming.

2. Remove from heat, then add the teabag to steep.

3. Let the milk cool in the refrigerator with the tea bag for about 30 minutes and then remove the teabag, squeezing gently to release all the flavor.

4. Place the milk, apple, and ice in a blender and blend until smooth.

5. Pour into 2 glasses and serve.

Nutrition:

- **Calories:** 88kcal **Fat:** 1g

- **Carbohydrates:** 19g

- **Phosphorus:** 74mg

- **Potassium:** 92mg

- **Sodium:** 47mg **Protein:** 1g

2. Watermelon-Raspberry Smoothie

Preparation time: 10 minutes. **Cooking time:** 0 minutes. **Servings:** 2

Ingredients:

- ½ cup boiled, cooled, and shredded red cabbage

- 1 cup diced watermelon ½ cup fresh raspberries 1 cup ice

Directions:

1. Put the cabbage in a blender and pulse for 2 minutes or until it is finely chopped.

2. Add the watermelon and raspberries and pulse for about 1 minute or until very well combined.

3. Add the ice and blend until very thick and smooth.

4. Pour into 2 glasses and serve.

Dialysis modification: The watermelon can be reduced by ½ cup to decrease potassium per serving by 50 mg.

Nutrition:

- **Calories:** 47kcal **Fat:** 0g **Carbohydrates:** 11g

- **Phosphorus:** 30mg **Potassium:** 197mg **Sodium:** 4mg

- **Protein:** 1g

3. Festive Berry Parfait

Preparation time: 1 hour and 20 minutes.

Cooking time: 0 minutes.

Servings: 4

Ingredients:

- 1 cup vanilla rice milk, at room temperature

- ½ cup plain cream cheese, at room temperature

- 1 tablespoon granulated sugar

- ½ teaspoon ground cinnamon

- 1 cup crumbled Meringue Cookies (<u>here</u>)

- 2 cups fresh blueberries

- 1 cup sliced fresh strawberries

Directions:

1. Whisk together the milk, cream cheese, sugar, and cinnamon until smooth in a small bowl,

2. Into 4 (6-ounce) glasses, spoon ¼ cup of crumbled cookie in the bottom of each.

3. Spoon ¼ cup of the cream cheese mixture on top of the cookies.

4. Top the cream cheese with ¼ cup of the berries.

5. Repeat in each cup with the cookies, cream cheese mixture, and berries.

6. Chill in the refrigerator for 1 hour and serve.

Nutrition:

- **Calories:** 243kcal **Fat:** 11g

- **Carbohydrates:** 33g

- **Phosphorus:** 84mg

- **Potassium:** 189mg

- **Sodium:** 145mg **Protein:** 4g

4. Chorizo and Egg Tortilla

Preparation: 10 minutes. **Cooking:** 13 minutes. **Servings:** 1 tortilla

Ingredients:

- 1 flour tortilla, about 6-inches 1/3 cup chorizo meat, chopped

- 1 egg

Directions:

1. Take a medium-sized skillet pan, place it over medium heat.

2. When it is hot, add chorizo and cook for 5 to 8 minutes until done.

3. When the meat has cooked, drain the excess fat, whisk an egg, pour it into the pan, stir until combined, and cook for 3 minutes, or until eggs have cooked.

4. Spoon egg onto the tortilla and then serve.

Nutrition:

- **Calories: 223 Cholesterol: 211ml Fat: 11g**

- **Net Carbs: 13.5g Protein: 16g Sodium: 317mg**

- **Carbohydrates: 15g**

- **Phosphorus: 232mg**

- **Fiber: 1.5g**

5. Corn Pudding

Preparation time: 10 minutes.

Cooking time: 40 minutes.

Servings: 6

Ingredients:

- Unsalted butter, for greasing the baking dish

- 2 tablespoons all-purpose flour

- ½ teaspoon Ener-G baking soda substitute

- 3 eggs

- ¾ cup unsweetened rice milk, at room temperature

- 3 tablespoons unsalted butter, melted

- 2 tablespoons light sour cream

- 2 tablespoons granulated sugar

- 2 cups frozen corn kernels, thawed

Directions:

1. Preheat the oven to 350°F.

2. Somehow grease an 8-by-8-inch baking dish with butter; set aside.

3. In a small bowl, mix the flour and baking soda substitute; set aside.

4. In a medium bowl, whisk together the eggs, rice milk, butter, sour cream, and sugar.

5. Stir the flour mixture into the egg mixture until smooth.

6. Add the corn to the batter and stir until very well mixed.

7. Spoon the batter into the baking dish and bake for about 40 minutes or until the pudding is set.

8. Let the pudding cool for about 15 minutes and serve warm.

Nutrition:

- **Calories:** 175

- **Fat:** 10g

- **Carbohydrates:** 19g

- **Phosphorus:** 111mg

- **Potassium:** 170mg

- **Sodium:** 62mg

- **Protein:** 5g

6. Rhubarb Bread Pudding

Preparation time: 15 minutes.

Cooking time: 50 minutes.

Servings: 6

Ingredients:

- Unsalted butter

- 3 eggs

- 1½ cups unsweetened rice milk

- ½ cup granulated sugar

- 1 tablespoon cornstarch

- 1 vanilla bean, split

- 10 thick pieces of white bread

- 2 cups chopped fresh rhubarb

Directions:

1. Preheat the oven to 350ºF.

2. In a bowl, whisk the eggs, sugar, rice milk, and cornstarch.

3. Scrape the vanilla seeds into the milk mixture and whisk to blend.

4. Place the bread in the egg combination and stir to coat the bread totally.

5. Add the chopped rhubarb and stir to combine.

6. Allow the bread and egg mixture to be the marinade for 30 minutes.

7. Spoon the combination, put it in the arranged baking dish, conceal it with aluminum foil, and then bake for 40 minutes.

8. Bare the bread pudding, then bake for an extra 10 minutes or up until the pudding is golden brown and set.

9. Serve the dish warm.

Dialysis modification: Decrease the rhubarb to 1 cup to bring the potassium to less than 150mg per serving. Or omit the rhubarb completely to bring the potassium to less than 75mg per serving. The bread pudding is delicious without the rhubarb, but it will be less tart.

Nutrition:

- **Calories:** 197kcal **Fat:** 4g

- **Carbohydrates:** 35g

- **Phosphorus:** 109mg

- **Potassium:** 192mg

- **Sodium:** 159mg

- **Protein:** 6g

Chapter 5:

Lunch

7. Aromatic Carrot Cream

Preparation time: 15 minutes.

Cooking time: 25 minutes.

Servings: 4

Ingredients:

- 1 tablespoon olive oil

- ½ sweet onion, chopped

- 2 teaspoons fresh ginger, peeled and grated

- 1 teaspoon fresh garlic, minced

- 4 cups water

- 3 carrots, chopped

- 1 teaspoon ground turmeric

- ½ cup coconut milk

Directions:

1. Heat the olive oil into a big pan over medium-high heat.

2. Add the onion, garlic and ginger. Softly cook for about 3 minutes until softened.

3. Include the water, turmeric and carrots. Softly cook for about 20 minutes (until the carrots are softened).

4. Blend the soup, adding coconut milk until creamy.

5. Serve and enjoy!

Nutrition:

- **Calories:** 112kcal **Fat:** 10g

- **Cholesterol:** 0mg **Carbohydrates:** 8g

- **Sugar:** 5g

- **Fiber:** 2g

- **Protein:** 2g

- **Sodium:** 35mg

- **Calcium:** 32mg

- **Phosphorus:** 59mg

- **Potassium:** 241mg

8. Mushrooms Velvet Soup

Preparation time: 40 minutes.

Cooking time: 40 minutes.

Servings: 6

Ingredients:

- 1 teaspoon olive oil

- ½ teaspoon fresh ground black pepper

- 3 medium (85grams) shallots, diced

- 2 stalks (80 grams) celery, chopped

- 1 clove garlic, diced

- 12-ounces cremini mushrooms, sliced

- 5 tablespoons flour

- 4 cups low sodium vegetable stock, divided

- 3 sprigs fresh thyme

- 2 bay leaves

- ½ cup regular yogurt

Directions:

1. Heat oil in a large pan.

2. Add ground pepper, shallots and celery; cook over medium-high heat.

3. Sauté for 2 minutes until golden.

4. Add garlic and stir.

5. Include the sliced mushrooms. Stir and cook until the mushrooms give out their liquid.

6. Sprawl the flour on the mushrooms and toast for about 2 min.

7. Add one cup of hot stock, thyme sprigs, and bay leaves. Stir and add the second cup of stock

8. Stir until well combined. Add the remaining cups of stock.

9. Slowly cook for 15 minutes. Take out bay leaves and thyme sprigs.

10. Blend until the mixture is smooth.

11. Include the yogurt and stir well.

12. Slowly cook for 4 minutes.

13. Serve and enjoy!

Nutrition:

- **Calories:** 126kcal **Fat:** 8g **Cholesterol:** 0mg **Carbohydrate:** 14g

- **Sugar:** 4g **Fiber:** 2g **Protein:** 3g **Sodium:** 108mg

- **Calcium:** 55mg **Phosphorus:** 70mg **Potassium:** 298mg

9. Easy Lettuce Wraps

Preparation time: 15 minutes.

Cooking time: 0 minutes.

Servings: 4

Ingredients:

- 8 ounces cooked chicken, shredded

- 1 scallion, chopped

- ½ cup seedless red grapes halved

- 1 celery stalk, chopped

- ¼ cup mayonnaise

- A pinch of ground black pepper

- 4 large lettuce leaves

Directions:

1. In a mixing bowl, add the scallion, chicken, celery, grapes, and mayonnaise.

2. Stir well until incorporated.

3. Season with pepper.

4. Place the lettuce leaves onto serving plates.

5. Place the chicken salad onto the leaves.

6. Serve and enjoy!

Nutrition:

- **Calories:** 146kcal

- **Fat:** 5g

- **Cholesterol:** 35mg

- **Carbohydrates:** 8g

- **Sugar:** 4g **Fiber:** 0g

- **Protein:** 16g

- **Sodium:** 58mg

- **Calcium:** 18mg

- **Phosphorus:** 125mg

- **Potassium:** 212mg

10. Couscous and Sherry Vinaigrette

Preparation time: 10 minutes. **Cooking time:** 30 minutes. **Servings:** 6

Ingredients:

For sherry vinaigrette: (makes 2/3 cup):

- 2 tablespoons sherry vinegar ¼ cup lemon juice

- 1 clove garlic, pressed 1/3 cup olive oil

For roasted carrots, cranberries, and couscous:

- 1 medium onion, sliced 2 large carrots, sliced

- 2 tablespoons extra-virgin olive oil

- 2 cups pearl couscous

- 2 ½ to 3 cups no-sodium vegetable broth

- ½ cup dried cranberries ¼ cup Sherry vinaigrette

Directions:

For sherry vinaigrette:

1. Beat the vinegar with garlic and lemon juice.

2. Slowly whisk in olive oil.

3. Store refrigerated in a glass jar.

For carrots, cranberries, and couscous:

1. Preheat oven to 400°F.

2. Spray a baking dish with cooking spray (olive oil) and place the carrots and onions on it.

3. Roast the vegetables in the oven for about 20 minutes until starting to brown. Stir halfway cooking.

4. Heat the couscous in a pan over medium-high heat.

5. Toast the couscous until light brown (about 10 minutes). Stir well.

6. Check the package instructions for the amount of liquid needed for couscous.

7. Bring to a boil the added vegetable stock. Cover and reduce for about 10 minutes. The vegetable stock has to be absorbed.

8. In a mixing bowl, incorporate the couscous with the onions, carrots, cranberries, and sherry vinaigrette.

9. Serve and enjoy!

Nutrition:

- **Calories:** 365kcal **Fat:** 11g **Cholesterol:** 0mg

- **Carbohydrate:** 58g **ugar:** 11g **Fiber:** 4g

- **Protein:** 9g **Sodium:** 95mg **Calcium:** 41mg

- **Phosphorus:** 119mg

- **Potassium:** 264mg

Chapter 6:

Dinner

11. Chicken and Pasta Salad

Preparation time: 30 minutes.

Cooking time: 25 minutes.

Servings: 6

Ingredients:

Chicken Pasta Salad

- 6 ounces cooked chicken

- 3 cups pasta, spiral, cooked

- ½ green pepper, minced

- 1 ½ tablespoon. onion

- ½ cup celery

Garlic Mustard Vinaigrette

- 2 tablespoon cider Vinegar

- 2 teaspoon mustard, prepared

- ½ teaspoon white sugar

- 1 garlic clove, Minced

- 1/3 cup water

- 1/3 cup olive oil

- 2 teaspoon parmesan cheese, grated

- ½ teaspoon ground pepper

Directions:

1. In a little bowl, combine vinegar, mustard, sugar, garlic, and water; slowly race in oil.

2. Mix the Parmesan cheese.

3. Season with pepper.

4. Join 1/3 measure of dressing with Chicken Pasta Salad ingredients and chill.

Nutrition:

- **Calories:** 233kcal **Fat:** 12g **Fiber:** 6g

- **Carbs:** 25g

- **Protein:** 23g

12. Herbed Soup with Black Beans

Preparation time: 10 minutes.

Cooking time: 10 minutes.

Servings: 4

Ingredients:

- 1/3 cup Poblano pepper, charred, peeled, seeded and chopped

- 2 cups vegetable stock

- ¼ teaspoon cumin

- ½ teaspoon paprika

- ½ teaspoon dried oregano

- 2 teaspoon fresh garlic, minced

- 1 cup onion, small diced

- 1 tablespoon extra-virgin olive oil

- 1 (15-ounces) black beans, drain and rinse

Directions:

1. On medium fire, place a soup pot and heat oil.

2. Sauté onion until soft.

3. Add garlic, cook for 2 minutes.

4. Add the remaining ingredients and let simmer.

5. Once simmering, turn off the fire and transfer to a blender.

6. Puree ingredients until smooth.

Nutrition:

- **Calories:** 98kcal

- **Fat:** 21g

- **Fiber:** 10g

- **Carbs:** 20g

- **Protein:** 19g

13. Herbs and Lemony Roasted Chicken

Preparation time: 6 minutes.

Cooking time: 11 minutes.

Servings: 8

Ingredients:

- ½ teaspoon ground black pepper

- ½ teaspoon mustard powder

- ½ teaspoon salt

- 1(3-pounds) whole chicken

- 1 teaspoon garlic powder

- 2 lemons

- 2 tablespoon olive oil

- 2 teaspoon Italian seasoning

Directions:

1. In a small bowl, mix well black pepper, garlic powder, mustard powder, and salt.

2. Rinse chicken well and slice off giblets.

3. Place chicken and add 1 ½ teaspoon of seasoning made earlier inside the chicken and rub the remaining seasoning around the chicken in a greased baking dish.

4. Mix olive oil and juice from 2 lemons in a small bowl,

5. Drizzle over chicken.

6. Bake chicken in a preheated 350ºF oven until juices run clear, around 1 ½ hour.

7. Every once in a while, baste the chicken with its juices.

Nutrition:

- **Calories:** 188kcal

- **Fat:** 9g

- **Fiber:** 6g

- **Carbs:** 20g

- **Protein:** 45g

14. Ground Chicken & Peas Curry

Preparation time: 15 minutes.

Cooking time: 6–10 minutes.

Servings: 3–4

Ingredients:

- 3 tablespoons essential olive oil

- 2 bay leaves

- 2 onions, grinded to some paste

- ½ tablespoon garlic paste

- ½ tablespoon ginger paste

- 1 tablespoon ground cumin

- 1 tablespoon ground coriander

- 1 teaspoon ground turmeric

- 1 teaspoon red chili powder

- Salt, to taste

- 1-pound lean ground chicken

- 2 cups frozen peas

- 1½ cups water

- 1–2 teaspoons garam masala powder

Directions:

1. In a deep-frying pan, heat oil with medium heat.

2. Add bay leaves and sauté for approximately half a minute.

3. Add onion paste and sauté for approximately 3–4 minutes.

4. Add garlic and ginger paste and sauté for around 1–1½ minutes.

5. Add spices and cook, occasionally stirring, for about 3–4 minutes.

6. Stir in chicken and cook for about 4–5 minutes.

7. Stir in peas and water and bring to a boil on high heat.

8. Reduce the heat to low and simmer approximately 5–8 minutes or till the desired doneness.

9. Stir in garam masala and remove from heat.

10. Serve hot.

Nutrition:

- **Calories:** 450kcal **Fat:** 10g

- **Carbohydrates:** 19g

- **Fiber:** 6g

- **Protein:** 38g

Chapter 7:

Vegetables and Salads

15. Vegetable Masala

Preparation time: 10 minutes.

Cooking time: 18 minutes.

Servings: 4

Ingredients:

- 2 cups green beans, chopped

- 1 cup white mushroom, chopped

- 1 teaspoon minced garlic

- 1 teaspoon minced ginger

- 1 teaspoon chili flakes

- 1 tablespoon garam masala

- 1 tablespoon olive oil

- 1 teaspoon salt

Directions:

1. Line the tray with parchment and preheat the oven to 360°F.

2. Place the green beans and mushrooms in the tray.

3. Sprinkle the vegetables with chopped garlic and ginger, chili flakes, garam masala, olive oil, and salt.

4. Mix up well and transfer in the oven.

5. Cook vegetable masala for 18 minutes.

Nutrition:

- **Calories:** 60kcal **Fat:** 30.7g

- **Fiber:** 2.5g

- **Carbs:** 6.4g

- **Protein:** 2g

16. Fast Cabbage Cakes

Preparation time: 15 minutes.

Cooking time: 10 minutes.

Servings: 2

Ingredients:

- 1 cup cauliflower, shredded

- 1 egg, beaten

- 1 teaspoon salt

- 1 teaspoon ground black pepper

- 2 tablespoons almond flour

- 1 teaspoon olive oil

- 3 cups chopped cabbage

Directions:

1. Blend the shredded cabbage in the blender until you get cabbage rice.

2. Then, mix up cabbage rice with the egg, salt, ground black pepper, and almond flour.

3. Pour olive oil into the skillet and preheat it.

4. Then make the small cakes with the help of 2 spoons and place them in the hot oil.

5. Roast the cabbage cakes for 4 minutes from each side over medium-low heat.

Nutrition:

- **Calories:** 227kcal

- **Fat:** 18.6g

- **Fiber:** 4.5g

- **Carbs:** 9.5g

- **Protein:** 9.9g

17. Cilantro Chili Burgers

Preparation time: 10 minutes.

Cooking time: 15 minutes.

Servings: 3

Ingredients:

- 1 cup red cabbage
- 3 tablespoons almond flour
- 1 tablespoon cream cheese
- 1 ounces scallions, chopped
- ½ teaspoon salt
- ½ teaspoon chili powder
- ½ cup fresh cilantro

Directions:

1. Chop red cabbage roughly and transfer it in the blender.
2. Add fresh cilantro and blend the mixture until very smooth.
3. After this, transfer it to the bowl.
4. Add cream cheese, scallions, salt, chili powder, and almond flour.
5. Stir the mixture well.
6. Make 3 big burgers from the cabbage mixture or 6 small burgers.

7. Line the baking tray with baking paper.

8. Place the burgers in the tray.

9. Bake the cilantro burgers for 15 minutes at 360°F.

10. Flip the burgers onto another side after 8 minutes of cooking.

Nutrition:

- **Calories:** 182kcal

- **Fat**: 15.3g

- **Fiber:** 4.1g

- **Carbs:** 8.5g

- **Protein:** 6.8g

18. Jicama Noodles

Preparation time: 15 minutes.

Cooking time: 7 minutes.

Servings: 6

Ingredients:

- 1-pound jicama, peeled

- 2 tablespoons butter

- 1 teaspoon chili flakes

- 1 teaspoon salt

- ¾ cup of water

Directions:

1. Spiralize jicama with the help of a spiralizer and place in jicama spirals in the saucepan.

2. Add butter, chili flakes, and salt.

3. Then add water and preheat the ingredients until the butter is melted.

4. Mix it up well.

5. Close the lid and cook noodles for 4 minutes over medium heat.

6. Stir the jicama noodles well before transferring them to the serving plates.

Nutrition:

- **Calories:** 63kcal

- **Fat:** 3.9g

- **Fiber:** 3.7g

- **Carbs:** 6.7g

- **Protein:** 0.6g

19. Crack Slaw

Preparation time: 15 minutes.

Cooking time: 10 minutes.

Servings: 6

Ingredients:

- 1 cup cauliflower rice

- 1 tablespoon sriracha

- 1 teaspoon tahini paste

- 1 teaspoon sesame seeds

- 1 tablespoon lemon juice

- 1 teaspoon olive oil

- 1 teaspoon butter - ½ teaspoon salt

- 2 cups coleslaw

Directions:

1. Toss the butter in the skillet and melt it.

2. Add cauliflower rice and sprinkle it with sriracha and tahini paste. Mix up the vegetables and cook them for 10 minutes over medium heat. Stir them from time to time. When the cauliflower is cooked, transfer it to the big plate. Add coleslaw and stir gently.

3. Then sprinkle the salad with sesame seeds, lemon juice, olive oil, and salt.

4. Mix it up well.

Nutrition:

- **Calories:** 76kcal **Fat:** 5.8g

- Fiber: 0.6g Carbs: 6g Protein: 1.1g

20. egan Chili

Preparation time: 10 minutes.

Cooking time: 20 minutes.

Servings: 4

Ingredients:

- 1 cup cremini mushrooms, chopped

- 1 zucchini, chopped

- 1 bell pepper, diced

- 1 ounces celery stalk, chopped

- 1 teaspoon chili powder

- 1 teaspoon salt

- ½ teaspoon chili flakes

- ½ cup of water

- 1 tablespoon olive oil

- ½ teaspoon diced garlic

- ½ teaspoon ground black pepper

- 1 teaspoon of cocoa powder

- 2 ounces Cheddar cheese, grated

Directions:

1. Pour olive oil into the pan and preheat it.

2. Add chopped mushrooms and roast them for 5 minutes. Stir them from time to time.

3. After this, add chopped zucchini and bell pepper.

4. Sprinkle the vegetables with the chili powder, salt, chili flakes, diced garlic, and ground black pepper.

5. Stir the vegetables and cook them for 5 minutes more.

6. Bring the mixture to boil and add water and cocoa powder.

7. Then add celery stalk.

8. Mix up the chili well and close the lid.

9. Cook the chili for 10 minutes over medium-low heat.

10. Then transfer the cooked vegan chili to the bowls and top with the grated cheese.

Nutrition:

- **Calories:** 123kcal **Fat:** 8.6g

- **Fiber:** 2.3g

- **Carbs:** 7.6g

- **Protein:** 5.6g

21. Chow Mein

Preparation time: 10 minutes.

Cooking time: 10 minutes.

Servings: 6

Ingredients:

- 7 ounces kelp noodles

- 5 ounces broccoli florets

- 1 tablespoon tahini sauce

- ¼ teaspoon minced ginger

- 1 teaspoon Sriracha

- ½ teaspoon garlic powder

- 1 cup of water

Directions:

1. Boil water in a sauce pan.

2. Add broccoli and boil for 4 minutes over the high heat.

3. Then drain water into the bowl and chill it tills the room temperature.

4. Soak the kelp noodles in the "broccoli water."

5. Meanwhile, place tahini sauce, sriracha, minced ginger, and garlic in the saucepan.

6. Bring the mixture to a boil. Add oil if needed.

7. Then add broccoli and soaked noodles.

8. Add 3 tablespoons of "broccoli water."

9. Mix up the noodles and bring to boil.

10. Switch off the heat and transfer Chow Mein to the serving bowls.

Nutrition:

- **Calories:** 18kcal

- **Fat:** 0.8g

- **Fiber:** 0.7g

- **Carbs:** 2.8g

- **Protein:** 0.9g

22. Mushroom Tacos

Preparation time: 10 minutes.

Cooking time: 15 minutes.

Servings: 6

Ingredients:

- 6 collard greens leave

- 2 cups mushrooms, chopped

- 1 white onion, diced

- 1 tablespoon Taco seasoning

- 1 tablespoon coconut oil

- ½ teaspoon salt

- ¼ cup fresh parsley

- 1 tablespoon mayonnaise

Directions:

1. Put the coconut oil in the skillet and melt it.

2. Add chopped mushrooms and diced onion. Mix up the ingredients.

3. Close the lid and cook them for 10 minutes.

4. After this, sprinkle the vegetables with Taco seasoning, salt, and add fresh parsley.

5. Mix up the mixture and cook for 5 minutes more.

6. Then add mayonnaise and stir well.

7. Chill the mushroom mixture a little.

8. Fill the collard green leaves with the mushroom mixture and fold up them.

Nutrition:

- **Calories:** 52kcal **Fat:** 3.3g

- **Fiber:** 1.2g **Carbs:** 5.1g

- **Protein:** 1.4g

23. Lime and Chickpeas Salad

Preparation time: 10 minutes.

Cooking time: 0 minutes.

Servings: 4

Ingredients:

- 400 grams chickpeas, drained and rinsed

- ½ tablespoon lime juice

- 2 tablespoons olive oil

- 1 teaspoon cumin, ground

- Sea salt and black pepper

- ½ teaspoon chili flakes

Directions:

1. In a bowl, mix the chickpeas and the rest of the ingredients, toss and serve cold.

Nutrition:

- **Calories:** 240kcal **Fat:** 8.2g **Fiber:** 5.3g

- **Carbs:** 11.6g

- **Protein:** 12g

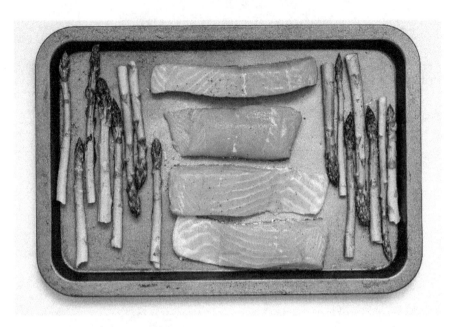

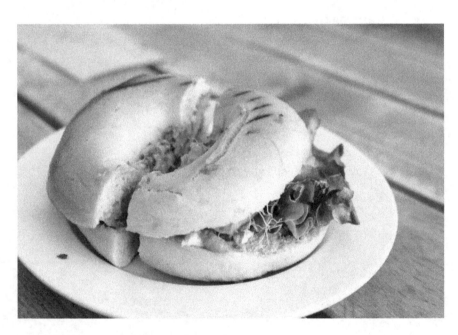

Chapter 8:

Seafood

24. Peppered Balsamic Cod

Preparation time: 10 minutes.

Cooking time: 2 hours.

Servings: 4

Ingredients:

- 1 1/2 pounds cod fillets

- 2 teaspoons olive oil

- 1 teaspoon lemon zest

- 1/2 teaspoon cracked black peppercorns

- 2 tablespoons balsamic vinegar, reduced to a syrup

Directions:

1. Cut a piece of foil large enough to wrap completely around the fish, or cut 4 smaller pieces to wrap the fish into individual packets.

Brush the foil with 1 teaspoon of the oil. Arrange the fish in the center of the foil and brush with the remaining oil. Season evenly with the lemon zest and pepper. Drizzle with the balsamic vinegar. Fold the foil completely around the fish and crimp the edges to seal the package(s).

2. Set the package in the slow cooker, cover with a lid, cook over high heat for 2 hours, or until the fish is cooked.

3. Serve at once.

Nutrition:

- **Calories: 201kcal Total fat: 5g**

- **Saturated fat: 1g**

- **Cholesterol: 101mg**

- **Sodium: 121mg**

- **Total carbohydrates: 1g;**

- **Dietary fiber: 1g;**

- **Protein: 39g;**

- **Sugars: 1g**

25. Seafood Gumbo

Preparation time: 25 minutes.

Cooking time: 5 hours.

Servings: 6

Ingredients:

- 2 teaspoons olive oil

- 1/4 cup minced turkey ham (low sodium)

- 2 stalks celery, sliced

- 1 medium onion, sliced

- 1 green bell pepper, chopped

- 2 cloves garlic, minced

- 2 cups chicken broth (low sodium)

- 400 grams diced tomatoes

- 1 teaspoon Worcestershire sauce

- 1/4 teaspoon kosher salt

- 1 teaspoon dried thyme

- 1-pound shrimp (16/20), cleaned

- 1-pound fresh or frozen crabmeat picked to remove cartilage

- 1 (10-ounce) package frozen okra, thawed

Directions:

1. Heat the oil in a sauté pan over medium-high heat. Add the ham and cook until crisp.

2. Transfer the ham to a slow cooker.

3. Add the celery, onion, green pepper, and garlic to the sauté pan and cook over medium heat, frequently stirring, until the vegetables are tender, about 10 minutes. Transfer to the cooker and add the broth, tomatoes, juices, Worcestershire, salt, and thyme.

4. Cover and cook over low heat for 4 hours. Add the shrimp, crabmeat, and okra, and cook over high heat or 20 minutes or until the shrimp is bright pink and firm.

5. Serve at once in heated soup bowls.

Nutrition:

- **Saturated fat:** 3g **Cholesterol:** 207mg **Sodium:** 313mg

- **Total carbohydrates:** 16g

- **Dietary fiber:** 5g **Protein:** 22g

- **Sugars:** 2g **Calories:** 155kcal

- **Total fat:** 5g

26. Salmon Chowder with Corn

Preparation time: 10 minutes.

Cooking time: 4 hours.

Servings: 4

Ingredients:

- 1 tablespoon butter

- 1 onion, finely chopped

- 1 clove garlic, minced

- 2 teaspoons dill weed

- Freshly ground black pepper

- 3 tablespoons all-purpose flour

- 2 cups chicken broth (low sodium)

- 2 cups milk 1 1/2 cups of corn kernels

- 12 ounces salmon fillet, cut into chunks

- 1 teaspoon grated lemon zest 3 tablespoons lemon juice

Directions:

1. Melt the butter on medium heat. Add the onion, garlic, dill, and a pinch of pepper; sauté, frequently stirring, until the onion is tender.

2. Add the flour and stir until thick and pasty, about 2 minutes.

3. Whisk in the broth until there are no lumps, then stir in the milk, and bring to a simmer.

4. Pour into the slow cooker and add the corn.

5. Cover with a lid and cook over low heat for 4 hours.

6. Stir in the salmon, replace the lid, cook over low heat for 20 minutes, or until the salmon is cooked (145°F) and very hot.

7. Stir in the lemon zest and season to taste with lemon juice and additional pepper.

8. Serve in heated soup bowls.

Nutrition:

- **Calories:** 391kcal **Total fat:** 18g

- **Saturated fat:** 9g

- **Cholesterol:** 94mg

- **Sodium:** 320mg

- **Total carbohydrates:** 39g

- **Dietary fiber:** 7g

- **Protein:** 37g

- **Sugars:** 17g

27. Mediterranean Fish Stew

Preparation time: 15 minutes.

Cooking time: 4 hours.

Servings: 6

Ingredients:

- 1 onion, sliced

- 1 leek, white and light green portion, sliced thin

- 4 cloves garlic, minced

- 1/2 cup dry white wine

- 1/4 cup water 4 bay leaves

- 1/2 teaspoon cracked black peppercorns

- 1 1/2 pounds haddock fillets

- 12 ounces shrimp (16/20), peeled and deveined

- 2 teaspoons extra-virgin olive oil for serving

- 2 tablespoons chopped parsley, flat-leaf

Directions:

1. Make a bed of the onion, leek, and garlic in the slow cooker. Add the wine and water to the cooker. Scatter the bay leaves and peppercorns on top.

2. Cover the cooker and cook over high heat for 2 hours. Add the fish and the shrimp, replace the cover, and cook over high heat for an additional 2 hours or until the fish is well cooked, and the shrimps are bright pink and opaque. Remove and discard the bay leaves.

3. Serve the fish and shrimp in heated soup bowls topped with the cooking liquid and vegetables. Drizzle with olive oil and garnish with parsley.

Nutrition:

- **Calories:** 207kcal

- **Total fat:** 4g

- **Saturated fat:** 0g

- **Cholesterol:** 168mg

- **Sodium:** 536mg

- **Total carbohydrates:** 5g

- **Dietary fiber:** 1g

- **Protein:** 32g

- **Sugars:** 0g

28. Sweet and Sour Shrimp

Preparation time: 10 minutes.

Cooking time: 5.5 hours.

Servings 3–4

Ingredients:

- 1 cup Chinese pea pods, thawed

- 400 grams pineapple chunks

- 2 tablespoons cornstarch

- 3 tablespoon sugar

- 1 cup chicken stock (see recipe)

- ½ cup reserved pineapple juice

- 1 tablespoon low-sodium soy sauce

- ½ teaspoon ground ginger

- 1-pound large cooked shrimp

- 2 tablespoon cider vinegar

- 1 cup of rice, cooked

Directions:

1. Place the pea pods and pineapple in a 4 to 6-quart slow cooker.

2. Blend the cornstarch and sugar with the chicken stock and pineapple juice and heat in a small saucepan until thickened.

3. Pour only the sauce into the slow cooker and add the ginger and soy sauce.

4. Cover and cook over low heat for 3 to 4 hours.

5. Add the shrimp and vinegar and cook for a further 15 minutes.

6. Serve with the hot cooked rice.

Nutrition:

- **Calories:** 395kcal

- **Fat:** 2g

- **Carbs:** 61g

- **Protein:** 33g

- **Fiber:** 5g

- **Potassium:** 796mg

- **Sodium:** 215 mg

Chapter 9:

Meat and Poultry

29. Shish Kebabs

Preparatlon time: 40 minutes.

Cooking time: 30 minutes.

Servings: 6

Ingredients:

- 1/2 cup olive oil

- 1/2 cup white vinegar

- 1/4 teaspoon garlic powder

- 1/2 teaspoon oregano

- 1/4 teaspoon black pepper

- 1 1/2 pounds beef sirloin, cubed

- 2 onions, sliced

- 2 green bell peppers, sliced

- 1 red bell pepper, sliced

Directions:

1. Combine oil, vinegar, garlic powder, oregano, and pepper in a bowl.

2. Soak the beef cubes in the marinade for 30 minutes.

3. Thread beef cubes and vegetables into the skewers. Grill for 30 minutes.

Nutrition:

- **Calories:** 358kcal **Protein:** 26g

- **Carbohydrates:** 5g **Fat:** 26g

- **Cholesterol:** 80mg **Sodium:** 60mg

- **Potassium:** 458mg **Phosphorus:** 217mg

- **Calcium:** 25mg **Fiber:** 1.4g

30. Tunisian Spiced Chicken

Preparation time: 10 minutes.

Cooking time: 40 minutes.

Servings: 4

Ingredients:

- 1 tablespoon olive oil

- 12 ounces boneless skinless chicken thighs

- ¼ small sweet onion, chopped

- 1 tablespoon grated peeled fresh ginger

- 2 teaspoons minced garlic

- 1 teaspoon paprika

- 1 teaspoon ground coriander

- ½ teaspoon ground cumin

- ¼ teaspoon ground turmeric

- ¼ teaspoon ground allspice

- ¾ cup basmati rice

- 1½ cups water

- 2 tablespoons chopped fresh cilantro

Directions:

1. In medium heat, heat the olive oil.

2. Brown the chicken on both sides 6 minutes total. Transfer to a plate.

3. In the skillet, add the onion, ginger, and garlic and sauté until softened, about 3 minutes.

4. Stir in the paprika, coriander, cumin, turmeric, allspice, and rice and mix well to coat the rice with the spices.

5. Add the water and the chicken, and bring the mixture to a boil. Reduce the heat to low, then cover the skillet. Simmer until the liquid is absorbed and the chicken is well cooked.

6. Garnish with the cilantro, and serve hot.

Nutrition:

- **Calories:** 265kcal **Total fat:** 7g

- **Saturated fat:** 1g **Cholesterol:** 70mg

- **Sodium:** 74mg **Carbohydrates:** 29g

- **Fiber:** 1g **Phosphorus:** 189mg

- **Potassium:** 264mg **Protein:** 19g

31. Crispy Fried Chicken

Preparation time: 15 minutes.

Cooking time: 30 minutes.

Servings: 4

Ingredients:

- ½ cup all-purpose flour

- 2 eggs, beaten

- ½ cup Italian seasoned bread crumbs

- ¼ teaspoon smoked paprika

- 12 ounces boneless skinless chicken thighs

- Pinch freshly ground pepper

- Olive oil cooking spray

Directions:

1. Preheat the oven to 350°F.

2. On a plate, place the flour, the eggs in a shallow bowl. Put the bread crumbs and paprika on another plate. Line the three dishes in a row.

3. Season a piece of chicken with pepper, dredge it first in the flour, then the egg, then the bread crumbs until the chicken is completely coated. Repeat for the remaining chicken.

4. On a baking sheet, arrange the chicken and coat lightly with cooking spray.

5. Bake until the chicken is well cooked, browned, and crispy, about 30 minutes.

6. Serve hot.

Nutrition:

- **Calories:** 246kcal

- **Total fat:** 7g

- **Saturated fat:** 2g

- **Cholesterol:** 175mg

- **Sodium:** 206mg

- **Carbohydrates:** 22g

- **Fiber:** 1g

- **Phosphorus:** 218mg

- **Potassium:** 261mg

- **Protein:** 23g

32. Tandoori Chicken

Preparation time: 15 minutes (plus 1-hour marinating time).

Cooking time: 30 minutes.

Servings: 4

Ingredients:

- 6 tablespoons plain yogurt

- 1 tablespoon freshly squeezed lemon juice

- 2 teaspoons grated peeled fresh ginger

- 2 teaspoons garam masala

- 1½ teaspoons curry powder

- 1 teaspoon honey

- 1 teaspoon minced garlic

- ½ teaspoon paprika

- Pinch cayenne pepper

- 4 (3-ounce) boneless skinless chicken breasts

Directions:

1. Whisk together the yogurt, lemon juice, ginger, garam masala, curry powder, honey, garlic, paprika, and cayenne pepper until well blended.

2. Add the chicken breasts to the mixture, and turn to coat. Cover and place the bowl in the refrigerator for at least 1 hour, or up to 12 hours, to marinate.

3. Preheat the oven to 400°F.

4. Remove from the marinade, and place them in a 9-by-9-inch baking dish.

5. Bake until the chicken is well cooked, turning once, about 30 minutes.

6. Serve hot.

Nutrition:

- **Calories:** 108kcal **Total fat:** 2g

- **Saturated fat:** 1g

- **Cholesterol:** 51mg

- **Sodium:** 61mg

- **Carbohydrates:** 2g

- **Fiber:** 0g

- **Phosphorus:** 159mg

- **Potassium:** 220mg

- **Protein:** 22g

33. Cauliflower-Topped Shepherd's Pie

Preparation time: 15 minutes.

Cooking time: 40 minutes.

Servings: 6

Ingredients:

- ½ head cauliflower, cut into florets

- 2 tablespoons unsalted butter, at room temperature

- 12 ounces extra-lean ground beef

- ½ small sweet onion, diced

- 2 teaspoons minced garlic

- 1 carrot, diced and parboiled until fork-tender

- 1 teaspoon chopped thyme

- ¼ teaspoon freshly ground black pepper

Directions:

1. Preheat the oven to 375°F.

2. Bring to a boil water in a saucepan.

3. Add the cauliflower, and blanch until tender, about 6 minutes.

4. Drain the cauliflower and mash with the butter until fluffy. Set it aside.

5. Brown the beef over high heat for about 6 minutes.

6. Sauté onion and garlic until softened, about 3 minutes.

7. Stir in the carrot and thyme.

8. Season with the pepper. Transfer the beef mixture to a 9-by-9-inch baking dish.

9. Top with the mashed cauliflower, and bake until bubbly, about 25 minutes.

10. Serve hot.

Nutrition:

- **Calories:** 128kcal **Total fat:** 7g

- **Saturated fat:** 4g **Cholesterol:** 45mg

- **Sodium:** 52mg **Carbohydrates:** 4g

- **Fiber:** 1g **Phosphorus:** 130mg

- **Potassium:** 341mg **Protein:** 13g

34. Salisbury Steak

Preparation time: 15 minutes.

Cooking time: 25 minutes.

Servings: 4

Ingredients:

- 12 ounces lean ground beef

- 1 small sweet onion, finely chopped

- ½ red bell pepper, seeded and finely chopped

- 1 teaspoon minced garlic

- 1 egg, beaten

- ½ teaspoon chopped fresh thyme

- ¼ teaspoon freshly ground black pepper

- 1 teaspoon olive oil

- ½ cup sodium-free beef stock, divided

- 1 tablespoon cornstarch

Directions:

1. Mix the beef, onion, bell pepper, garlic, egg, thyme, and pepper.

2. Form the mixtures into patties about ½ inch thick.

3. Heat the olive oil; brown the patties on both sides, about 6 minute's total.

4. Add ¼ cup of stock to the skillet and simmer for 15 minutes, turning the patties once.

5. Remove the patties to a plate, cover, and set aside.

6. Whisk the cornstarch into the remaining ¼ cup of stock, and add the mixture to the skillet.

7. Simmer, whisking, until the sauce thickens to a gravy consistency.

8. Serve the patties topped with the sauce.

Nutrition:

- **Calories:** 153kcal **Total fat:** 7g

- **Saturated fat:** 2g

- **Cholesterol:** 105mg

- **Sodium:** 117mg

- **Carbohydrates:** 2g

- **Fiber:** 0g

- **Phosphorus:** 193mg

- **Potassium:** 361mg

- **Protein:** 20g

35. Mouthwatering Beef and Chili Stew

Preparation time: 15 minutes.**Cooking:** 7 hours.**Servings:** 6

Ingredients:

- 1/2 medium red onion, 1/2 tablespoon. vegetable oil

- 10oz of flat-cut beef brisket, whole

- ½ cup low sodium stock ¾ cup water

- ½ tablespoon honey tablespoon chili powder

- ½ teaspoon smoked paprika ½ teaspoon dried thyme

- 1 teaspoon black pepper

- 1 tablespoon cornstarch

Directions:

1. Throw the sliced onion into the slow cooker first.

2. Add a splash of oil to a large hot skillet and briefly seal the beef on all sides.

3. Remove the beef from the skillet and place it in the slow cooker.

4. Add the stock, water, honey, and spices to the same skillet you cooked the beef.

5. Loosen the browned bits from the bottom of the pan with a spatula. (Hint: These brown bits at the bottom are called the fond).

6. Allow the juice to simmer until the volume is reduced by about half.

7. Pour the juice over beef in the slow cooker.

8. Cook (low) for approx. 7 hours on a slow cooker.

9. Take the beef out of the slow cooker and onto a platter.

10. Shred-it with two forks.

11. Pour the juice into a pan. Bring to a simmer.

12. Whisk the cornstarch with two tablespoons of water.

13. Add to the juice and cook until slightly thickened.

14. For a thicker sauce, simmer and reduce the juice a bit more before adding cornstarch.

15. Pour the sauce on the meat and serve.

Nutrition:

- **Calories:** 128kcal **Protein:** 13g

- **Carbohydrates:** 6g **Fat:** 6g

- **Cholesterol:** 39mg **Sodium:** 228mg

- **Potassium:** 202mg **Phosphorus:** 119mg

- **Calcium:** 16mg **Fiber:** 1g

36. Beef and Three Pepper Stew

Preparation time: 15 minutes.

Cooking time: 6 hours.

Servings: 6

Ingredients:

- 10 ounces of flat-cut beef brisket, whole

- 1 teaspoon of dried thyme

- 1 teaspoon of black pepper

- 1 clove garlic

- ½ cup of green onion, thinly sliced

- ½ cup low-sodium chicken stock

- 2 cups water

- 1 large green bell pepper, sliced

- 1 large red bell pepper, sliced

- 1 large yellow bell pepper, sliced

- 1 large red onion, sliced

Directions:

1. Combine the beef, thyme, pepper, garlic, green onion, stock, and water in a slow cooker.

2. Leave it all to cook over high heat for 4–5 hours until tender.

3. Remove the beef from the slow cooker and let it cool.

4. Shred the beef and remove excess fat.

5. Place the shredded beef back into the slow cooker.

6. Add the sliced peppers and the onion.

7. Cook (high) for 45 minutes or until the vegetables are tender.

Nutrition:

- **Calories:** 132kcal **Protein:** 14g

- **Carbohydrates:** 9g **Fat:** 5g

- **Cholesterol:** 39mg **Sodium:** 179mg

- **Potassium:** 390mg **Phosphorus:** 141mg

- **Calcium:** 33mg

- **Fiber:** 2g

Chapter 10:

Soups and Stews

37. Coney Dog Sauce

Preparation time: 20 minutes.

Cooking time: 4 hours.

Servings: 8

Ingredients:

- 1 pound lean ground beef

- 2 cup low-sodium tomato sauce

- ½ cup water

- 1½ tablespoon low-sodium Worcestershire sauce

- ¼ cup onion, finely chopped

- 1 tablespoon ground mustard

- ½ teaspoon garlic powder

- ½ teaspoon freshly ground black pepper

- ½ teaspoon chili powder

- ¼ teaspoon cayenne pepper

Directions:

1. Brown the ground beef in a large heavy-based frying pan.

2. Add the cooked ground beef along with all other ingredients to a 4 to 6-quart slow cooker.

3. Cover and cook over low heat for 4 hours.

4. Serve as a topping with low-sodium hot dogs.

Nutrition:

- **Calories:** 112kcal

- **Fat:** 4g

- **Carbs:** 5g

- **Protein:** 12g

- **Fiber:** 1g

- **Potassium:** 210mg

- **Sodium:** 83mg

38. Curried Cauliflower Soup

Preparation time: 20 minutes.

Cooking time: 30 minutes.

Servings: 6

Ingredients:

- 1 teaspoon unsalted butter

- 1 small sweet onion, chopped

- 2 teaspoons minced garlic

- 1 small head cauliflower

- 3 cups water, or more to cover the cauliflower

- 2 teaspoons curry powder

- ½ cup light sour cream

- 3 tablespoons chopped fresh cilantro

Directions:

1. In a large saucepan, heat the butter over medium-high heat and sauté the onion and garlic for about 3 minutes or until softened. Add the cauliflower, water, and curry powder.

2. Bring the soup to a boil, then lessen the heat to low and simmer for about 20 minutes or until the cauliflower is tender. Pour the

soup into a food processor and purée until it is smooth and creamy (or use a large bowl and a handheld immersion blender).

3. Transfer the soup back into a saucepan and stir in the sour cream and cilantro. Heat the soup on medium-low for about 5 minutes or until it is well heated.

Nutrition:

- **Calories:** 33kcal **Fat:** 2g

- **Carbs:** 4g

- **Phosphorus:** 30mg

- **Potassium:** 167mg

- **Sodium:** 22mg

- **Protein:** 1g

39. Cream of Watercress Soup

Preparation time: 15 minutes.

Cooking time: 1 hour 15 minutes.

Servings: 4

Ingredients:

- 6 garlic cloves

- ½ teaspoon olive oil

- 1 teaspoon unsalted butter

- ½ sweet onion, chopped

- 4 cups chopped watercress

- ¼ cup chopped fresh parsley

- 3 cups of water

- ¼ cup heavy cream

- 1 tablespoon freshly squeezed lemon juice

- Freshly ground black pepper

Directions:

1. Pre-heat the oven to 400°F. Set your garlic on a sheet of foil. Drizzle with olive oil and fold the foil into a little packet. Place the packet

on a pie plate and roast the garlic for about 20 minutes or very soft.

2. Switch off the oven and set your garlic to cool. Add your butter to melt in a saucepan on medium heat. Sauté the onion for about 4 minutes or until soft. Add the watercress and parsley; sauté 5 minutes. Stir in the water and roasted garlic pulp. Allow boiling, then switch the heat to low.

3. Simmer the soup for about 20 minutes or until the vegetables are soft. Cool the soup for about 5 minutes, then purée in batches in a food processor (or use a large bowl and a handheld immersion blender), along with the heavy cream.

4. Transfer the soup to the pot, and set over low heat until it is well warmed. Add the lemon juice and season with pepper.

Nutrition:

- **Calories:** 97kcal **Fat:** 8g

- **Carbs:** 5g **Phosphorus:** 46mg

- **Potassium:** 198mg

- **Sodium:** 23mg

- **Protein:** 2g

Chapter 11:

Desserts

40. Chocolate Beet Cake

Preparation time: 10 minutes.

Cooking time: 50 minutes.

Servings: 12

Ingredients:

- 3 cups grated beets

- 1/4 cup canola oil

- 4 eggs

- 4 ounces unsweetened chocolate

- 2 teaspoon Phosphorus-free baking powder

- 2 cups all-purpose flour 1 cup sugar

Directions:

1. Set your oven to 325°F. Grease two 8-inch cake pans.

2. Mix the baking powder, flour, and sugar. Set aside.

3. Slice up the chocolate as excellently as you can and melt using a double boiler. A microwave can also be used, but don't let it burn.

4. Allow it to cool, and then mix in the oil and eggs.

5. Mix all of the wet ingredients into the flour mixture and combine everything until well mixed.

6. Fold the beets in and pour the batter into the cake pans.

7. Let them bake for 40 to 50 minutes. To know it's done, the toothpick should come out clean when inserted into the cake.

8. Remove from the oven and allow them to cool.

9. Once cool, invert over a plate to remove.

10. It is great when served with whipped cream and fresh berries. Enjoy!

Nutrition:

- **Calories:** 270

- **Protein:** 6g

- **Sodium:** 109mg

- **Potassium:** 299mg

- **Phosphorus:** 111mg

Chapter 12:

Meal Plan (15 Days)

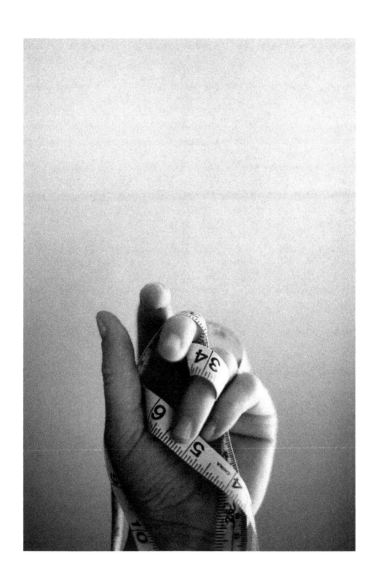

Day #	Breakfast	Lunch	Dinner
Day 1	Mixed Vegetable Barley	Cajun Crab	Ground Beef and Rice Soup
Day 2	Spicy Sesame Tofu	Salad with Lemon Dressing	Beef Curry Delight
Day 3	Egg Fried Rice	Shrimp Salsa	Herbs and Lemony Roasted Chicken
Day 4	Vegetable Rice Casserole	Eggplant Salad	Salad Greens with Roasted Beets
Day 5	Savory Muffins with Protein	Mediterranean Pork	Seafood Casserole
Day 6	Italian Apple Fritters	Ground beef and Bell Peppers	Baked Flounder
Day 7	Blueberry Smoothie Bowl	Almond Chicken	Beef Chili
Day 8	Egg white Pepper Omelets	Aromatic Carrot Cream	Shrimp Paella
Day 9	Chicken Egg Rolls	Mushroom velvet soup	Salmon & Pesto Salad
Day 10	Mexican style Burritos	Mushroom Pork chops	Cod & Green Bean Risotto
Day 11	Sweet Pancakes	Caramelized Pork Chops	Chicken Mandarin Salad
Day 12	Egg and Veggie muffins	Juicy Salmon Dish	Chicken and Pasta Salad
Day 13	Apple-chai Smoothie	Platter-O-Brussels	Chicken Stew
Day 14	Cheesy scrambled eggs with fresh herbs	Blackberry Chicken Wings	Tomato Stuffed Portobello Caps
Day 15	Festive berry parfait	Spaghetti with Pesto	Ground Pork with Water Chestnuts

Conclusion

Managing chronic kidney disease (CKD) requires lifestyle adjustments, but it might help to know that you're not alone. Over 31 million people in the United States are diagnosed with malfunctions of their kidneys or are battling kidney disease. As a registered dietitian (RD) with extensive experience assisting patients in taking control of their kidney disease, I have helped patients manage the physical symptoms associated with this disease and cope with the emotional toll that this life change can take. Without knowing what the future holds, uncertainty, fear, depression, and anxiety can be common. It may even feel like dialysis is inevitable, and you may be asking yourself if it is worth the time or effort to try and manage this stage of the disease or if it's even possible to delay the progression. As an expert in this field, I can assure you it is not just possible; it's yours to achieve—only 1 in 50 diagnosed with CKD end up on dialysis. So together and with the right tools, we can work to delay and ultimately prevent end-stage renal disease and dialysis. Success is earned through diet modifications and lifestyle changes. Using simple, manageable strategies, I have watched firsthand as my patients empowered themselves with knowledge. They have gone on to lead full, productive, and happy lives, continuing to work, play, and enjoy spending time with their loved ones—just the way it should be!

CPSIA information can be obtained
at www.ICGtesting.com
Printed in the USA
BVHW091429030521
606339BV00006B/968